THE DIABETES ALERT

Winning The Battle Against Blood Sugar

By

Mary J. Douglas

Table of Contents

Introduction

Karen was a woman living with diabetes, and she was determined to make the best of it. From the time she was diagnosed, she took charge of her condition with strength and resilience, believing that she could still make a full life despite her diagnosis. She soon found that with the right amount of care and attention, she could manage her condition and lead a productive, fulfilling life.

Karen devoted her time to learning as much as she could about her condition, researching the latest news and treatments, and joining support groups. She found that being around others who were dealing with the same issues made her feel less alone, and gave her a sense of community. She also made lifestyle changes to improve her health, such as eating a nutritious diet, exercising regularly, and monitoring her blood sugar levels.

Karen was determined to remain positive, and to make a difference in her community. She volunteered her time to diabetes organizations, and attended fundraising events to help raise awareness about the condition. She also shared her story with others, and encouraged them to take charge of their condition as well.

Karen's story of resilience and determination is one of courage and hope. Her journey with diabetes is an inspiration to others, and her example highlights that Diabetes is a chronic condition characterized by high levels of sugar in the blood. It is caused when the body does not produce enough insulin, or when the body cannot effectively use the insulin it produces. Diabetes is a serious condition that can lead to a range of health complications if left untreated. People with diabetes need to manage their condition by making lifestyle changes, such as eating healthy and exercising regularly, as well as taking medication and monitoring their blood sugar levels. With proper management, it is possible to reduce the risk of developing complications related to diabetes.

This introduction provides an overview of diabetes, including its causes and health implications. It also outlines the importance of managing diabetes and the steps that can be taken to reduce the risk of complications.

Chapter 1

Understanding Diabetes

Diabetes is a chronic, metabolic disorder in which the body cannot properly regulate levels of glucose (blood sugar) in the blood. This is caused when the body either does not produce enough insulin, or cannot use the insulin it produces effectively. When not managed properly, diabetes can cause a number of serious health issues including heart disease, stroke, kidney disease, vision problems, and nerve damage.

Diabetes is generally managed with a combination of lifestyle modifications such as eating a balanced diet, maintaining a healthy body weight, and exercising regularly. In some cases, medication and/or insulin injections may be needed to help the body regulate glucose levels. It is important for people with diabetes to monitor their blood sugar closely, and to regularly visit the doctor for check ups. With proper management, individuals with diabetes can lead healthy, active lives.

Types Of Diabetes

Diabetes is in two major forms namely Type 1 and Type 2. Other rare types of diabetes include gestational diabetes, latent autoimmune diabetes of adults (LADA), and monogenic diabetes.

- **Type 1 Diabetes**

Type 1 diabetes is a disease in which the body's immune system attacks and destroys the cells in the pancreas that produce insulin. This results in an inability to produce enough insulin, which is necessary to regulate blood sugar levels. As a result, people with type 1 diabetes must take insulin injections every day in order to survive. It is normally detected in children and youths, although it can occur at any age.

There is currently no cure for type 1 diabetes, but research is ongoing to try and find ways to prevent, treat, and even reverse the condition. In the meantime, people with type 1 diabetes must take good care of themselves to ensure that they can manage their condition and stay healthy.

- **Type 2 Diabetes**

Type 2 diabetes is chronic disease that affects how the body processes glucose, or blood sugar. It is the most common type of diabetes, affecting around 90 percent of people with the disease. People with type 2 diabetes are at higher risk for heart disease, stroke, kidney disease, and other health problems.
The principal source of type 2 diabetes is an unhealthy way of living. This includes being overweight, eating a diet high in processed foods, and not getting enough physical activity. These factors can lead to insulin resistance, which is when the body doesn't respond properly to insulin. As a result, glucose builds up in the blood instead of being used for energy.

- **Gestational Diabetes**

Gestational diabetes is a type of diabetes that takes in the course of pregnancy. It affects about 4% of all pregnant women in the United States. It is caused by changes in the hormones produced by the placenta, which can interfere with the body's ability to use and make insulin. Without enough insulin, the body is unable to use the sugar in the blood, leading to high blood sugar levels.

Gestational diabetes can have grave outcome for both the mother and the baby. Uncontrolled gestational diabetes can lead to large babies, preterm delivery, and an increased risk of caesarean section. The baby can also be at risk of low blood sugar, jaundice, and respiratory problems.

Women with gestational diabetes should follow a healthy diet and exercise regularly to keep their blood sugar levels in check. It is important to monitor blood sugar levels closely to make sure that they are within a safe range. In some cases, insulin injections may be needed to help control blood sugar levels.

Women with gestational diabetes should also receive regular prenatal care throughout their pregnancies. Close monitoring of the baby's growth and development is important to make sure that the baby is growing and developing normally.

Gestational diabetes usually resolves after pregnancy, but women who have had gestational diabetes are at an increased risk of developing type 2 diabetes later in life. Regular check-ups and lifestyle modifications can help reduce this risk.

Prediabetes

Prediabetes is a condition in which the quantity of blood sugar is higher than normal, but not high enough to be classified as diabetes. It is a precursor to type 2 diabetes and is typically diagnosed when a person has an A1C level of 5.7-6.4%. Prediabetes is a growing health concern, impacting an estimated 84 million Americans. The most common risk factors for prediabetes are obesity, being over 45 years old, having a family history of diabetes, being physically inactive, and having high blood pressure or cholesterol.

Prediabetes can be managed through lifestyle changes, such as eating a healthy diet, increasing physical activity, and maintaining a healthy weight. In some cases, medication may be prescribed to help control blood sugar levels. It is important to take prediabetes seriously, as it is a precursor to type 2 diabetes and can lead to serious health complications if left untreated.

Chapter 2

Causes Of Diabetes

Too much glucose circulating in your bloodstream causes diabetes, regardless of the type. However, the reason why your blood glucose levels are high differs depending on the type of diabetes. Causes of diabetes include:

- **Genetics**

Genetics play a key part in the development of diabetes. Genes can influence the risk of developing type 1 and type 2 diabetes. Genes can also affect how the body responds to insulin, which is an important factor in managing diabetes.

Type 1 diabetes is an autoimmune disorder where the body's own immune system attacks and destroys the beta cells in the pancreas that produce insulin. It is known to be caused by a fusion of genetic and environmental factors. Several genes have been identified that are associated with an increased risk of developing type 1 diabetes.

Type 2 diabetes is a complex disorder with multiple genetic and environmental factors playing a role. There are several genes that are associated with an increased risk of developing type 2 diabetes. These genes can influence the body's response to insulin and the development of insulin resistance, which is an important factor in the development of type 2 diabetes.

People with a family history of diabetes should be especially mindful of their lifestyle choices to reduce their risk of developing diabetes.

- **Obesity**

Obesity and diabetes are closely linked. Obesity increases the risk of developing type 2 diabetes, and people with diabetes are more likely to be obese. Obesity can cause insulin resistance, which is when the body's cells don't respond properly to insulin, leading to high blood sugar levels. People who are overweight or obese are also more likely to have other conditions associated with diabetes, such as high blood pressure and high cholesterol. In order to reduce the risk of developing diabetes, it is important to maintain a healthy weight and be physically active. Eating a balanced diet, limiting calorie intake, avoiding processed and sugary foods, and reducing stress can also help to reduce the dangers of diabetes.

- **Sedentary Lifestyle**

Sedentary way of life is a principal risk factor for developing type 2 diabetes. People who are physically inactive are more likely to gain weight, which can lead to insulin resistance and an increased risk of diabetes. People who sit for long periods of time without engaging in physical activity have an increased risk of developing type 2 diabetes, even if they maintain a healthy weight. This is because a sedentary lifestyle can decrease the body's ability to properly use insulin, which can lead to elevated blood sugar levels. Additionally, people who are physically inactive have higher levels of inflammation in the body, which can also contribute to diabetes. Therefore, to reduce the risk of developing type 2 diabetes, it is important to maintain an active lifestyle and engage in regular physical activity.

- **Unhealthy Diet And Diabetes**

Unhealthy dietary habits are a major risk factor for developing type 2 diabetes. Eating a diet that is high in refined carbohydrates, saturated fat, and added sugars can cause a person to become overweight or obese, which in turn increases the risk of developing diabetes. Eating a diet that is low in nutrients and high in unhealthy foods can also increase the risk of developing diabetes, as well as other chronic health conditions such as heart disease and stroke. Eating a balanced diet that is rich in fruits, vegetables, whole grains, and lean proteins can help reduce the risk of developing diabetes. Additionally, engaging in regular physical activity can help lower the risk of diabetes.

- **Stress And Diabetes**

Stress can have a major impact on a person's ability to manage their diabetes. It can interfere with the body's ability to process glucose, resulting in higher blood sugar levels. It can also lead to unhealthy behaviors, such as overeating, which can result in weight gain and further complicate diabetes management. In addition, stress can cause people with diabetes to skip meals or take their medication inconsistently, leading to further complications. To help manage stress, people with diabetes should make time for relaxation, exercise, and talking to their healthcare provider about managing their stress.

- **Pregnancy**

Pregnancy and diabetes can be a complicated and risky combination. Diabetes can cause serious health problems for both a pregnant woman and her baby. Women with diabetes should work closely with their healthcare team to manage their diabetes and reduce the risks associated with diabetes during pregnancy. Women with diabetes should have their blood sugar levels monitored before, during and after pregnancy. Women with diabetes should also follow a healthy diet, exercise regularly, and take medications as prescribed. Women with diabetes should also consult with their healthcare team regarding their risk of developing other complications, such as high blood pressure, during pregnancy.

In addition to managing their diabetes, pregnant women with diabetes should be aware of the potential risks to their unborn baby. These include an increased risk of birth defects, low birth weight, preterm delivery, and stillbirth. Women with diabetes should also be aware of the potential risks associated with delivering a large baby, such as shoulder dystocia.

Pregnancy can be a difficult and complicated journey, but with careful planning and management, women with diabetes can have healthy pregnancies and healthy babies.

- **Age**

Age is a strong risk factor for diabetes. The risk of developing diabetes increases with age. In fact, the risk is approximately twofold for adults aged 45-64 years and fivefold for adults aged 65 and older compared to adults aged 18-44 years. Additionally, people aged 65 and older are more likely to have type 2 diabetes than any other age group.

Aging can increase the risk of diabetes because as people age, their bodies become less able to produce and use insulin. In addition, age-related changes in the body's cells can make people more resistant to the effects of insulin. Other risk factors associated with age-related diabetes include obesity, physical inactivity, and certain medical conditions, such as high blood pressure or high cholesterol.

Age-related diabetes can be managed with lifestyle modifications, such as eating a healthy diet, engaging in regular physical activity, and maintaining a healthy weight. Medications may also be prescribed to help manage diabetes.

- **Race**

Race and ethnicity can have a significant impact on the risk of developing diabetes. African Americans, Native Americans, Asian Americans, and Hispanic Americans are all more likely to develop diabetes than non-Hispanic whites. African Americans are twice as likely to develop diabetes than non-Hispanic whites, and Native Americans, Asian Americans, and Hispanic Americans are 1.5 times more likely to develop diabetes than non-Hispanic whites. Additionally, African Americans, Native Americans, and Hispanic Americans are more likely than non-Hispanic whites to develop complications from diabetes, including kidney failure, amputations, and blindness.

There are numerous potential explanations for why race and ethnicity are associated with a higher risk of developing diabetes. These explanations include genetic susceptibilities, environmental exposures, and access to healthcare. It is also thought that racial and ethnic minorities may be more exposed to risk factors for diabetes, such as a lower socio-economic status, poorer nutrition, and less access to healthcare.

Given the significant impact of race and ethnicity on the risk of developing diabetes, it is important for

healthcare providers to be aware of this connection and to provide culturally sensitive care to all patients. Additionally, public health initiatives should focus on reducing disparities in access to healthcare and improving health
literacy in under-served populations

Chapter 3

Symptoms Of Diabetes

Symptoms of diabetes can vary greatly from person to person and can range from mild to severe. The popular symptoms of diabetes include:

- **Increased thirst**

Increased thirst in diabetics is a common symptom that can be caused by high blood sugar levels. High blood sugar levels can cause fluid to be pulled out of the tissues, leading to dehydration. This can cause the body to signal to the brain that it needs more fluids, resulting in increased thirst. Other symptoms of dehydration can include fatigue, headaches, dark-colored urine, and dry mouth. If a person with diabetes is experiencing increased thirst, they should drink plenty of fluids and monitor their blood sugar levels. They should also consult their doctor to determine the cause of their increased thirst and to ensure that their diabetes is well-controlled.

- **Frequent Urination**

Frequent urination in diabetics is a common symptom of diabetes caused by elevated blood sugar levels. Diabetes causes the body to produce more urine to try to rid the body of the excess glucose. As a result, people with diabetes may have to urinate more frequently, especially during the night.

- **Extreme Hunger**

If you have diabetes, you may be at risk of experiencing extreme hunger. This is because diabetes can disrupt normal communication between your brain and your body, making it difficult for your body to recognize when it has had enough food. This can lead to episodes of extreme hunger, which can be difficult to manage.

To help manage extreme hunger, it is important to monitor your blood sugar levels and adhere to your diabetes treatment plan. Eating regular meals and snacks throughout the day, as well as limiting foods that are high in sugar and carbohydrates, can help you manage your blood sugar levels. Additionally, incorporating exercise into your daily routine and speaking with your doctor about medications or other treatments can help you better manage your diabetes and extreme hunger.

- **Unexplained Weight Loss**

Unexplained weight loss is a common symptom of diabetes, particularly type 1 diabetes. People with diabetes may lose weight due to lack of insulin in the body, leading to the body being unable to convert food into energy properly. People with diabetes may also experience increased appetite and thirst due to high blood sugar levels, leading to weight loss. Other symptoms of diabetes such as frequent urination, fatigue, blurred vision, and slow healing of cuts and bruises may also be present. It is important to talk to your doctor if you are experiencing unexplained weight loss to determine the underlying cause and make sure you receive appropriate treatment.

- **Fatigue**

Fatigue is a common symptom of diabetes. It is caused by high blood sugar levels, which can lead to dehydration and a lack of energy. Other factors that may contribute to fatigue in people with diabetes include poor blood sugar control, a lack of regular physical activity, and depression. To help manage fatigue, it is important to maintain good blood sugar control, get regular physical activity, and eat a healthy, balanced diet. In some cases, medications and supplements may be used to help manage fatigue.

- **Blurry Vision**

Yes, blurry vision can be a sign of diabetes. High blood sugar levels can cause changes in the shape of the lens of the eye, which in turn can cause blurry vision. Other symptoms of diabetes include frequent urination, excessive thirst, unexplained weight loss, fatigue, and slow healing of wounds. If you are experiencing any of these symptoms, it is important to make an appointment with your doctor as soon as possible.

- **Slow healing sores**

Diabetics often have slow healing sores due to their impaired circulation and nerve damage. To help heal slow healing sores, diabetics should:

- Keep the area clean by washing it with mild soap and water and applying an antibiotic ointment.

- Change the dressing regularly.

Apply a moist compress to the wound to help speed healing.

- Elevate the affected area to reduce swelling.

- Ask their doctor about taking a vitamin supplement to help their wound heal.

- Control and manage their blood sugar levels

- Avoid smoking, as it can slow healing.

- Follow the doctor's instructions for wound care

- **Frequent Infections**

People with diabetes are at a much higher risk of developing infections than those without diabetes. This is because diabetes can weaken the immune system, making the body less able to fight off bacteria and viruses. Frequent infections that can occur in people with diabetes include urinary tract infections, skin infections, gum infections, and yeast infections. It is important to practice good hygiene and to monitor blood sugar levels regularly to help reduce the risk of infection. Additionally, people with diabetes should see their healthcare provider regularly to assess their risk of infection and receive preventive care.

- **Tingling Or Numbness In The Hands Or Feet**

Tingling or numbness in the hands or feet, known as neuropathy, is a common symptom of diabetes. It occurs when high blood sugar levels cause nerve damage in the hands, leading to a loss of sensation. Symptoms may include a feeling of pins and needles, burning, or numbness in the hands and fingers. Treatment for neuropathy typically includes medications and lifestyle changes to help keep blood glucose levels under control.

- **Dark Patches Of Skin**

Dark patches of skin in diabetics is a common symptom of a condition called diabetic dermopathy.

This condition occurs due to changes in the small blood vessels of the skin, causing them to enlarge and become more easily visible. The patches are typically found on the front of the legs and appear as circles or ovals that are either lighter or darker than the surrounding skin. The patches can be itchy and scaly, but they are usually painless. If you notice any dark patches on your skin, it is important to talk to your doctor to determine the cause.

- **Vaginal Yeast Infection**

Women living with diabetes have a higher risk of developing vaginal yeast infections. This is because high levels of glucose in the blood can cause the fungus that causes yeast infections (Candida) to grow faster. Symptoms of a vaginal yeast infection can include itching, burning, and a thick white discharge.

If you have diabetes and suspect you have a yeast infection, it is important to see your doctor. He or she can diagnose the infection and prescribe a course of treatment. This may include an oral antifungal medication, an antifungal cream, or suppository. It is also important to keep your blood sugar levels in check to prevent further yeast infections. Adopting a healthy diet and avoiding sugary foods and drinks can help to reduce your risk of yeast infections.

Diagnosis Of Diabetes

Diabetes is typically diagnosed through a combination of blood tests and a physical exam. A blood test for diabetes is used to measure the amount of glucose (sugar) in the blood, which may be an indicator of diabetes. Other tests may include a urine test to check for the presence of glucose, an HbA1c test, which measures blood glucose levels over the past three months, and an oral glucose tolerance test, which measures the body's ability to process glucose. Your doctor may also perform a physical exam to look for signs and symptoms of diabetes, such as excessive thirst, frequent urination, and weight loss.

- **A1C Test**

The A1C test is a blood test used to measure average blood sugar levels over the past 2-3 months. It is a key tool for managing diabetes and is recommended for all people with diabetes at least twice a year. The A1C test measures the amount of haemoglobin (a protein in red blood cells) that has glucose attached to it. The higher the A1C level, the higher the average blood sugar level has been over the past 2-3 months. A normal A1C level is below 5.7%, while an A1C of 6.5% or higher on two separate tests indicates diabetes. The A1C test is a quick and easy way to get an overall picture of your blood sugar control. It can help you and your doctor determine the best treatment plan for you and make sure that your diabetes is under control.

- **Random Blood Sugar Test.**

Blood sugar values are revealed in milligrams of sugar per deciliter (mg/dL) or millimoles of sugar per liter (mmol/L) of blood. No matter when you has your last meal, a level of 200 mg/dL (11.1 mmol/L) or higher suggests diabetes, especially if you also have symptoms of diabetes, such as frequent urination and extreme thirst.

- **Fasting Blood Sugar Test.**

A sample of blood is taken on an empty stomach before you eat anything. Results are interpreted as follows:
Below 100 mg/dL (5.6 mmol/L) is considered healthy.

100 to 125 mg/dL (5.6 to 6.9 mmol/L) is diagnosed as prediabetes.
126 mg/dL (7 mmol/L) or higher on two separate tests is diagnosed as diabetes.

Oral Glucose Tolerance Test.

This procedure is seldom used than the others, it is mostly used during pregnancy. You must not eat for a certain amount of time and then drink a sugary liquid at your health care provider's office. For two hours your blood sugar levels will be tested

Intermittently. Results are interpreted as follows:
Below 140 mg/dL (7.8 mmol/L) after two hours is considered healthy.
140 to 199 mg/dL (7.8 mmol/L and 11.0 mmol/L) is diagnosed as prediabetes.
200 mg/dL (11.1 mmol/L) or higher after two hours suggests diabetes.

Chapter 4

Treatments

- **Diet**

A healthy diet is an important part of diabetes treatment. Eating a balanced diet that is low in fat, salt, and sugar can help control blood glucose levels, reduce the risk of diabetes complications, and improve overall health. Eating a variety of foods from all food groups, including plenty of fruits, vegetables, and whole grains, can help to ensure a balanced diet. Planning meals in advance and keeping a food diary can help to manage diabetes. Additionally, limiting the intake of sugary foods and beverages, such as soda and candy, can help to reduce blood glucose

Working with a doctor or dietitian to create an individualised plan and setting realistic goals will be helpful.

- **Exercise**

Exercise is an important part of diabetes treatment. It can help lower blood sugar levels and improve your overall health. Exercise can also help improve your body's sensitivity to insulin and increase your energy levels. Regular physical activity is also important for managing diabetes and achieving a healthy weight. Do at least 30 minutes of moderate physical activity at least four days of the week. Activities such as walking, jogging, swimming, and biking can all help to burn calories and promote your well-being. Tips for exercising with diabetes:

- Start slowly. If you're new to exercising, start with gentle activities like walking or swimming.

- Choose activities that you enjoy. Exercise doesn't have to be a chore. Choose routines that are fun and makes you happy.

- Check your blood sugar before and after every workout. This will help you see how exercise affects your blood sugar levels.

- Stay hydrated. Always bring a bottle of water with you when you exercise.

- Wear the right shoes. Make sure you have shoes that are comfortable and provide support.

- Take breaks. Don't push yourself too hard. Take breaks as needed.

- Talk to your doctor. Ask your doctor for advice and any necessary precautions when it comes to exercising with diabetes.

- **Weight loss**

Losing weight is a very important part of diabetes treatment. Excess weight is associated with an increased risk of developing type 2 diabetes, and losing even a few pounds can help reduce the risk. Additionally, losing weight can help people with diabetes better manage their blood sugar levels and improve their overall health.

When it comes to weight loss for people with diabetes, the goal should be to lose fat, not muscle. A healthy diet and regular physical activity are important for achieving this goal. Eating a balanced diet that focuses on vegetables, fruits, and whole grains is important for maintaining a healthy weight.

Additionally, limiting portion sizes, avoiding sugary and processed foods, and reducing calories can help promote weight loss.

Finally, it's important to talk to your doctor before beginning any weight loss program. They can help you draw a plan that will suit your individual needs and health goals.

- **Monitor Your Blood Sugar**

Monitoring your blood sugar level is an major role of managing diabetes. It helps you to understand how food, physical activity and medication affect your blood sugar levels. It is important to monitor your blood sugar levels regularly to ensure that they remain within a healthy range. You may want to check your blood sugar levels before meals, after meals, and at bedtime. You should also check your blood sugar levels if you experience any symptoms of low or high blood sugar. To monitor your blood sugar levels, you will need a glucose meter, test strips, and lancets.

When you check your blood sugar, make sure to record the results in a logbook. This will help your healthcare provider to follow your progress and make any necessary adjustments to your treatment plan. Your healthcare provider can also use the information from your logbook to determine if any lifestyle changes are necessary. It is important to keep track of your blood sugar levels and to follow up with your healthcare provider regularly.

Medications For Diabetes

- **Insulin**

Insulin is a medication used to treat people with diabetes. It helps to regulate the amount of sugar in the blood by allowing the body to use glucose from food as energy. It can also be used to help people with certain other medical conditions. It is usually taken as an injection, but some people may also use an insulin pump.

- **Sulfonylureas**

Sulfonylureas are oral medications that stimulate the pancreas to produce more insulin. These drugs are used to treat type 2 diabetes and are usually prescribed in combination with other medications. Common side effects include hypoglycemia, weight gain, nausea, and skin rash.

- **Metformin**

Metformin is administered orally and it's used treating type 2 diabetes. It works by lowering the quantity glucose produced by the liver and elevating the body's sensitivity to insulin. It also helps to lower blood glucose levels and improve the body's ability to use insulin more effectively. It may also help reduce the risk of cardiovascular disease, lower cholesterol levels, and reduce the risk of developing certain types of cancer. Metformin is usually taken once or twice a day with meals. It is typically prescribed in combination with lifestyle changes such as eating a healthy diet and exercising regularly.

- **Gliptins**

Gliptins are a class of medications used to treat type 2 diabetes. They work by increasing the body's sensitivity to insulin, which helps to lower blood sugar levels. Gliptins are typically taken in combination with other diabetes medications, such as metformin, and with lifestyle changes, such as diet and exercise.

- **Thiazolidinediones**

Thiazolidinediones (TZDs) are a class of antidiabetic drugs used to treat type 2 diabetes. They work by increasing the body's sensitivity to insulin, which helps the body better utilize insulin and glucose. TZDs also aid in reducing blood sugar levels by lowering the amount of glucose produced by the liver. TZDs can also help reduce cholesterol and triglyceride levels. Pioglitazone and Rosiglitazone are some examples of TZDs

- **Meglitinides**

Meglitinides are a class of drugs used to treat type 2 diabetes. They are used in combination with diet and exercise to help lower blood sugar levels. Meglitinides work by stimulating the body to produce more insulin, which helps move glucose out of the bloodstream and into the cells, where it can be used as energy. These drugs are taken orally and usually have a quick onset of action, usually within 30 minutes. Common side effects include weight gain, headache, and hypoglycemia.

- **Alpha-glucosidase**

Alpha-glucosidase is an enzyme that catalyzes the hydrolysis of the alpha-1,4 and alpha-1,6 glycosidic linkages in the polysaccharides and oligosaccharides. Alpha-glucosidase is involved in the digestion of carbohydrates in the small intestine, and it is also responsible for the breakdown of disaccharides such as maltose, sucrose and lactose. Inhibition of alpha-glucosidase can decrease the absorption of dietary carbohydrates and is thus used as a treatment for type 2 diabetes.

- **DPP-4 inhibitors**

DPP-4 inhibitors are a class of drugs used to treat type 2 diabetes, a condition in which the body does not produce or use insulin properly. These drugs work by blocking the action of an enzyme called dipeptidyl peptidase-4 (DPP-4), which breaks down peptides that signal the body to produce insulin. By blocking DPP-4, these drugs help to keep levels of insulin in the body at a higher level and help to control blood sugar levels. Examples of DPP-4 inhibitors include sitagliptin (Januvia), saxagliptin (Onglyza), linagliptin (Tradjenta), and alogliptin (Nesina).

Chapter 5

Prevention Of Diabetes

- **Eat A Healthy Diet**

Eating a balanced diet rich in whole grains, fruits and vegetables can help prevent type 2 diabetes. Include plenty of fiber, such as beans, legumes, nuts, and seeds. Eating lean proteins, such as fish, chicken, and lean beef, can also help.

- **Exercise Regularly**

Physical activity helps keep your blood sugar levels in check and helps your body use insulin more efficiently. Do a 30 minute moderate-intensity exercise most days of the week.

- **Maintain A Healthy Weight**

Obesity elevates your risk of developing type 2 diabetes. Maintaining a weight within the healthy range can help lower your risk.

- **Quit Smoking**

Tobacco inhalation increases your risk of developing type 2 diabetes. Quit smoking to reduce your risk of developing the condition.

- **Monitor Your Blood Sugar**

Regularly monitoring your blood sugar levels can help you stay on top of your diabetes and lower your risk of complications.

- **Manage Stress**

Stress can increase your risk of developing type 2 diabetes. Learning how to manage stress can help lower your risk.

- **Get Enough Sleep**

Sleep deprivation can increase your risk of developing type 2 diabetes. Get enough sleep get at least seven hours each night.

- **Regular Check-Ups**

Taking regular check-ups are important for maintaining good health. Regular check-ups help detect any problems early on, so that appropriate treatment can be provided. These check-ups should include a physical exam, blood tests, and other tests as recommended by a healthcare provider. In addition to physical exams, it's important to have regular screenings for things such as cholesterol levels, diabetes, and other health conditions. Regular check-ups also allow a doctor to keep track of any changes or developments in a person's health, so they can provide the most appropriate care.

Regular check-ups are important for everyone, regardless of age. However, it is especially important for people over the age of 40 and those with chronic health conditions. People with chronic health conditions may need more frequent check-ups and more in-depth tests. It is also important for pregnant women to have regular check-ups, as this can help detect any potential issues with the pregnancy.

Conclusion

In conclusion, this book has provided an in-depth look into the various aspects of diabetes. It has discussed the symptoms, diagnosis, and treatment of diabetes, as well as lifestyle changes and dietary adjustments that can help manage this chronic condition. It has also provided helpful tips for dealing with the emotional and psychological aspects of living with diabetes. We hope this book has helped to provide a better understanding of diabetes and its management. With the right knowledge and support, it is possible to live a healthy and active life with diabetes.

9 7 9 8 3 9 4 2 5 8 0 6 0